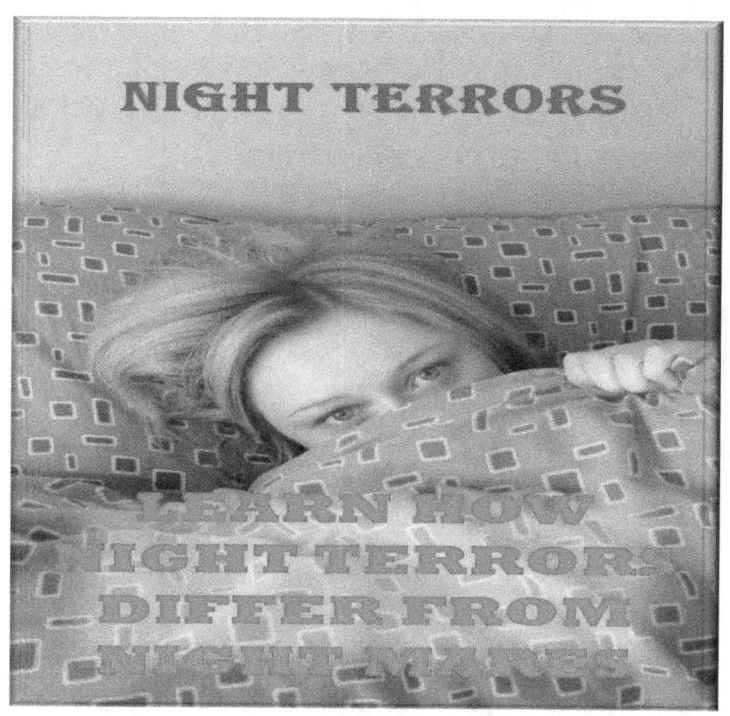

By Patricia A Carlisle

Introduction

I want to thank you and congratulate you for choosing the book, *"NIGHT TERRORS: LEARN HOW NIGHT TERRORS DIFFER FROM NIGHTMARES"*.

Dreams occur during the period of sleep called REM (Rapid Eye Movement), which is repeated three or four times a night.

A **nightmare** is a dream that takes place during REM sleep. But this dream causes intense feelings of fear, invincibility, terror, distress, or extreme anxiety. These feelings usually awake little babies dreaming nightmares, with total or partial remembrance of what they dreamed.

A **night terror** is an episode of extreme fear during sleep, with no remembrance of the dream itself. The child awakes screaming and crying, without knowing what he dreamed, being unable to say what scared him so badly and having a state of horror that is likely to persist even after apparently awake. Unlike nightmares, night terrors occur during non-REM sleep (dreamless sleep.) Children wake up sweating, with a rapid pulse and frightened. They are not aware of what is around them and don't respond to attempts of calming them. The crisis may last from 10, 15 or 30 minutes.

The good thing is that there are children who fall asleep immediately after the crisis ended. And most of the times, children don't remember what scared them in their sleep. But in rare cases they remember some fragmentary picture of the "dream".

It seems that many nightmares and night terrors occur more often in childhood. At child or at adult, these terrifying night-time experiences tend to occur in periods in which the individuals is uncertain, have emotional disorders, depression, feelings of guilt, the existence of unresolved psychological conflicts, or traumatic events.

These night terrors are occurring as a part of post-traumatic stress syndrome. There are a number of high emotional events that may disturb the children's sleep, and may go unnoticed by their parents. Examples of these emotional events are: loss of a loved object or favorite toy, a fight with another child at play, an injustice that he/she did, or someone has made to them. But the most emotional disrupt is hearing argues between parents.

There are children who suffer from serious psychological problems, which are the source of these nightmares. Psychotherapy may be the solution of solving these problems, but it is extremely important to know the child's and their family history. Even though nightmares and night terrors are considered normal events, common in development, but not mandatory, most times, they disappear in adolescence. Yet, if the occurrence frequency of these phenomena is high, then it requires expert evaluation.

Thanks again for choosing this book, I hope you enjoy it!

ABOUT THE AUTHOR
PATRICIA A. CARLISLE, MSW, CBT

Patricia Carlisle- a Master Social Worker and Cognitive Behavioral Therapist (CBT) gives out an expression of how important it is for an individual to take into consideration the concept of self-assessment to know what human, technical and conceptual skills they posses to perform or to achieve what they desire, or to deal with everyday life. However, every particular group of people has their own unique set of ideas, traditions and events including the frame of mind according to which people perform but there are many who faces problems and fail to maintain a healthy mind set affecting their behaviors and performance to those around them.

People like Patricia Carlisle are among those who have felt this urge of serving people and helping them out of their mental crisis towards a healthy life. She has experienced some close encounters in her personal life regarding mental health issues in her family and friends that has encouraged her to pursue this as her career.

Currently Patricia Carlisle is serving as a Certified On-Line Cognitive Behavioral Therapist with an extensive 15years of experience using Cognitive-Behavior Therapy Techniques. She envisions a world where everyone gets mental health treatment with no mental health stigma and to make it real she has already set up her own Holistic Measure Online Comprehensive Behavioral Healthcare Company after retiring from The Nord Center in The Partial Hospitalization Program (PHP) Dept for 5 years and Murtis H. Taylor Mental Health Center as a mental health counselor, psychological support technician and case manager for 10 years to emulsify her skills more professionally.

Along with this, she has wrote down her passion as a clinician in 25 or more short books to help individuals and families get their life back, freeing them of the restraints of negative thinking, anxiety and depression by using different approaches. She is highly appreciated among her clients for her flexibility and professionalism of dealing with them graciously. To reach her, make use of her direct website address: http://therapist2013.wix.com/e-therapy . As she is ready to inspire hope and contribute to health and well-being by providing the best online health care through comprehensive practice, education and research.

TABLE OF CONTENT

Chapter 1

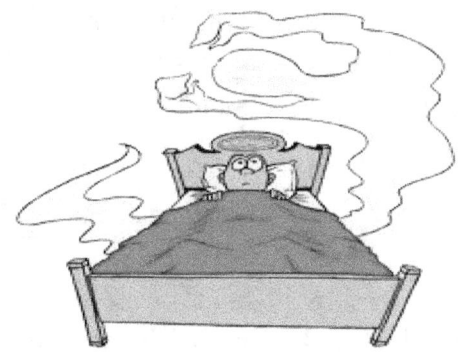

NIGHTMARES

Nightmares are defined as distressing dream that generally keep you awake. Many times the person experiencing the nightmare will feel anxiety, fear, depression, sadness or anger. These feelings are all commonly associated with nightmares. One of the most common themes of nightmares tends to be being chased by an unknown person however nightmares do come in a variety of themes.

Nightmares actually tend to be a part of adolescent development, as most children will have nightmares between the ages of three to eight. Adults experience nightmares at a lesser frequency with about 5-10% of adults having one nightmare a month. An occasional nightmare is nothing to be concerned about at any age.

They are experiences that can be very frightening and incredibly disturbing. The feeling when awoken is of relief, and the thought that it was only a bad dream nothing more. However, the feelings and images of these nightmares can frighten some people for the whole day or even for years.

Different Causes of Nightmares

What causes nightmares has been studied and discussed for thousands of years, and unfortunately even with the most modern technology the scientists haven't been able to come up with a precise answer for this question.

Physical illnesses such as fevers cause nightmares, as can rapid withdrawal of drugs, or by taking certain medications or drugs. Most nightmares experienced by little children tend to emerge when the child is struggling dealing with normal fears, or other childhood problems. Individuals that have undergone a traumatic event tend to experience nightmares.

Nightmares can be caused by physical conditions that affect health. Stress is one of the causes for nightmares. If someone is under extreme stress, nightmares are a way that Mother Nature finds to release all the pressure suffered by the dreamer.

Nightmares can also be caused from stress during the day such as difficulty at work, financial concerns, moving, or a pregnancy. There are also nightmares that affect people that are in no way related to their daytime activities. Many times these individuals are highly emotional, creative and sensitive.

Post-traumatic stress disorders can also cause the individual to have nightmares. This is where someone has been through some kind of event that caused emotional or physical trauma. The memories and feelings about that specific event can cause sleeping disorders, especially nightmares.

Worries are also a big trigger for nightmares. If someone is worried about something at a particular time then it is very likely they will have a nightmare around that time. Some people are classed as 'worriers'. With constant worrying about something they are the most affected ones as they are likely to heave regular nightmares.

Nightmares can also be genetic; studies showed that individuals with frequent nightmares have a family history of similar sleeping disturbances. Childhood is when nightmares are the most common, because this is a time of our emotional development when we all have to come to terms with, well, raw, primitive emotions such as aggression and rage.

The imbalance of our emotions can also cause us to have frequent nightmares. Primitive emotions such as rage and aggression, profound resentment, excessive fear, and an over competitive character may trigger frequent nightmares.

Nightmares can occur after losing a loved one, surgery, severe accident, or participating in combat. Many times the theme of the nightmare will relate back to the traumatic event.

Treatment

- o Write down your nightmare in as much detail as you can remember. Tell the whole story even if it is extremely scary.

- o Try to end the story of your nightmare with a happy ending. Do not include violence of any sort when writing the story. Keep it as peaceful and compassionate as you can. Don't forget that you are working with raw emotions, and trying to turn them into more refined emotions.

- o After you finish writing the new story, go through it in your head over and over again. You must do this every night right after you go to bed. Don't do anything in between as it will weaken this powerful technique. Do it when you go to bed, so you are not tempted to do things in between.

o Then do some relaxation exercises. You can choose anyone that you are comfortable with such a yoga, meditation, or breathing exercises.

o Treating the nightmare will depend on the cause of the nightmare. If drugs cause your nightmares then you should speak to your doctor. Therapy is an option if you or a family member is suffering from recurring nightmares. It is important to understand what your fear is and how to deal with it so you feel safe.

Chapter 2

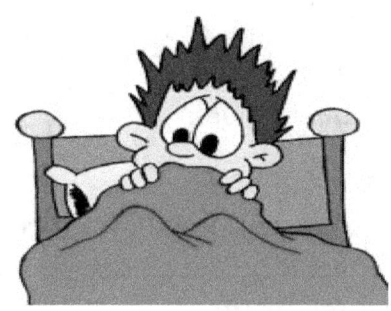

NIGHT TERROR

Night terrors are sleep disturbances in which a child may suddenly sit bolt upright in bed, cry scream, moan, and mumble and thrash about with her eyes wide open, but without being truly awake. Because they are caught in a sort of a twilight zone between being asleep and being awake, their unaware of your presence, and isn't likely to respond to anything you say or do. An episode can last anywhere from 2 to 40 minutes, and when it's over your child falls back to sleep abruptly with no memory of the incident.

What Causes Night Terrors

There's no definitive way to prevent night terrors because no one knows exactly what cause them. Night terrors can result from an erratic or insufficient sleep routine, or any type of sleep deprivation. They may be caused by stress experienced during the day, or over-tiredness. There is even some evidence that night terrors run in families. What is known is, on their own, night terrors do not mean a child has a psychological problem, or is even upset about something.

Those of you who have witnessed a child's night terror will know how they came to be named. The child wakes abruptly from sleep in a confused and very frightened state, showing physical signs of panic such as sweating, rapid breathing, and elevated heart rate. Often the child will thrash around, scream, appear very distressed, and seem unaware of their surroundings, or of your efforts to comfort them.

They may not even recognize you and this is because, even though their eyes are open, your child is actually still in a deep sleep state. These episodes can last for as long as forty minutes before the child returns to a restful sleep with no memory of the event the next day. Night terrors appear so frightening however that you as a parent are often left shocked and wide-eyed for considerably longer. It's important to reassure yourself that night terrors are common, and are not at all harmful for your child.

Night terrors sometimes run in families. They occur most often in the 2 to 7 year group, and more often in boys, although, can also occur in girls and in older children and even, rarely, in adults. Episodes seem to occur more frequently when children also have a sleep disorder such as obstructive sleep apnea.

Night terrors differ from nightmares and are not as common. Night terrors are episodes of arousal occurring during 'deep sleep' or 'slow wave sleep'. Because we get most of our deep sleep early in the night, episodes generally occur during the first third of the night.

In contrast, nightmares occur during rapid eye movement sleep (REM sleep or 'dream sleep') much later-generally in the early hours of the morning. Sometimes it's possible to identify triggers such as high fevers, being overtired, and emotional stress on the previous day. These are useful to consider since, for some children, addressing these triggers prevents further episodes.

In general, night terrors do not usually require further investigation or treatment, and there is no association between childhood night terrors and future mental health problems. Most often kids simply grow out of them as their sleep develops and matures. Night terrors are a horrible thing for both the person suffering from them, and the person who experiences them happening. If you see a loved one in a state in the middle of the night, when they are asleep, but have their eyes opened, can be very frightening. This is because you are unable to comfort them or calm them down. It seem to be more common in children than in adults. However, they usually last just a few minutes.

How Night Terrors Affect the Body

Rapid breathing usually occurs, the heart races, the sufferer will have a rapid pulse, and they will also start to sweat. The person who suffers from them will usually sits up in the bed in a state, maybe have their eyes open, and will take a while before they can be woken up.

The Danger Area

The person can become a danger to themselves, or others while having an episode. The person may jump out of bed, swing his arms and legs, and fight with anyone who tries to calm him. However, this is more common in adults than it is in children. The worst part of the whole thing is when you try to calm the person down they do not here you until the episode has passed.

Wakening

In children, when they wake up from the episode they will not remember it, but adults usually will remember something of the dream.

Sound

The night terror will result in the person screaming and crying, especially in children. They may shout and moan, and might mumble things that do not make sense at all.

Sight

The person may stare at nothing at all, or may stare directly at you (although they do not see you).

Long Term Effect

They are something most children grow out of. They are also really rare in adults. Medical intervention is only needed if the person dreads going to sleep due to the night terrors, if they are increasing in frequency, or if they result in someone getting hurt.

Chapter 3

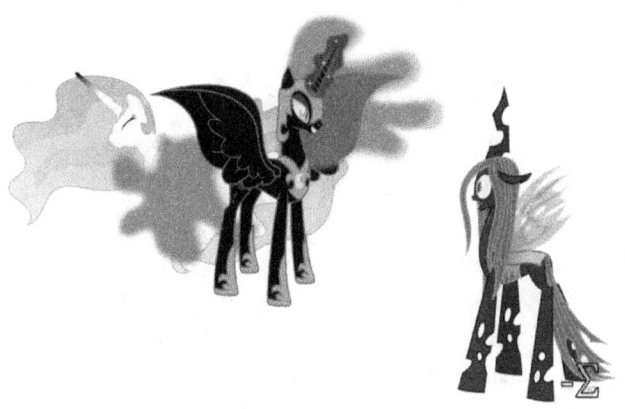

NIGHTMARES VS NIGHT TERRORS

One question sleep disorder suffers often ask is "Did I have a nightmare or a night terror? And what is the difference?" Night terrors & nightmares actually have a distinct difference from one another, and the scientific classifications between the two are clear.

Nightmares are likely to take place following a period of many hours of deep sleep. The victim remembers the dream- sometimes in exacting detail. This is one of the biggest differences between nightmare and night terrors: the night mare victim nearly always becomes aware that they experienced an intense dream after waking up or perhaps shortly thereafter. Although the nightmare itself could get a person directly out of bed, there's hardly ever any kind of thrashing about, or any physical movements that accompany the nightmare other than whimpers or perhaps some slight groans.

Once the nightmare sufferer awakens, he or she tends to remember the dream experience to have been fearful, although they may not be able to pinpoint exactly why. Quite often, the sleeper benefits from talking about the details of their nightmare with someone close to them.

However, if a person experiences nightmares consistently over a prolonged period of time, it could indicate a more serious sleeping problem-perhaps even an actual sleep disorder.

Night terrors, however, take place within the first couple of hours of sleep. When they strike, the sleeper responds with defending shouting which is almost always accompanied by intense thrashing in bed. Waking the sleeper up is very difficult, and the sleeper usually doesn't remember much of anything other than an overwhelming sensation, or perhaps an individual scene from their dream. In many cases, the victim doesn't remember anything at all.

Nightmares and night terrors develop during distinctly different periods of sleep. Young children who have experienced night terrors may also tend to walk in their sleep and/or discharge urine in bed. Nightmare sufferers, on the other hand, seldom experience these reactions, regardless of their age.

Compared to nightmares, scientists don't really have a good handle on what causes night terrors. More in-depth research is definitely needed to uncover the causes. Once puberty arrives, children generally stop experiencing them.

In adults, however, night terrors are commonly caused by stressful daytime situations and experiences. In cases such as this, a consultation with a doctor experienced in the field of sleep disorders would be highly recommended. Victims of both nightmares as well as night terrors can benefit from a consultation with a sleep disorder specialist.

Chapter 4

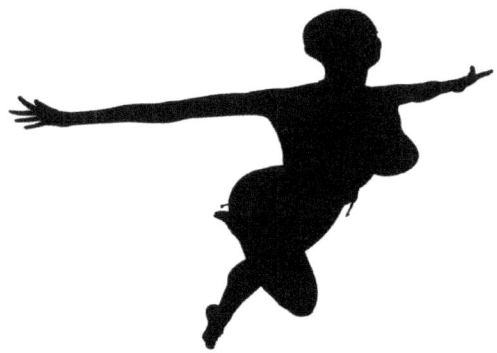

OVERCOMING NIGHTMARES THROUGH LUCID DREAMING

Nightmares can be defined as an unpleasant and frightening dream. They're completely harmless, but not something anyone wants to experience as they sleep. They can leave individuals scared, and even have the person traumatized; leaving them unable to sleep the next night in fear of it occurring again.

Just imagine yourself having the capability to put an end to a terrifying nightmare. Something that not many people can say they can do. Does that intrigue you? It sure intrigues me!

How to Stop Nightmares

The ability to become conscious through a dream is considered the most efficient way of escaping the harsh and brutal nightmares being endured. Yes, that's right; lucid dreams have been proven to prevent nightmares and enable an escape. It should also be noted that many current lucid dreamers are lucid on the basis of having a nightmare, only to come to the epiphany that it MUST be a dream.

Now that we've established that, let's discuss how this can happen, and how you can be well on your way to putting an end to your nightmares. The two techniques experts are talking about are commonly used by many professional and active lucid dreamers, and are able to be used by anyone in a lucid nightmare.

Learn How to Lucid Dream

Firstly, learning how to lucid dream is essential. This may seem obvious, but the first thing you must do to stop nightmares from happening is to be able experience these dreams. The lucid dream needs to be practiced in order to allow you to consciously act in your nightmares, which is of extreme importance to putting an end to nightmares. Once you have gained control of your dreams, and able to attain lucidity on a regular basis, you are one step closer to putting an end to nightmares you may face in the future. Please note that this step is crucial, and may be tedious to master.

Waking Up

For those of you who have mastered the art of achieving these dreams-congratulations. It's often difficult to achieve, but you've done it! Now, let's talk about waking up through the act of a lucid dream in order to stop nightmares.

Waking up is common practice through lucid dreaming to stop a nightmare. It has been done many times, and will continue to be practiced as it's an effective way to put an end to a nightmare. As soon as you enter lucidity within a nightmare, a way to wake yourself up is to simply shout "WAKE UP! As you blink hard in the dream. As a result, you will most likely come to an end with your nightmare, and can then proceed to go back to sleep, or whatever you feel like doing.

Confront the Nightmare

Even though the waking up method works, what you are not doing is confronting the nightmare, which can be done through a lucid dream. Given nightmares can be incredibly scary, it's no wonder why you'd want to wake up within an instant of being exposed to the nightmare. After all, you're only human! That being said, once you build up the courage within a lucid dream while experiencing a nightmare, confronts the nightmare and overcome what you fear. Ask for answers. Don't feel like you're completely helpless from the nightmare.

Although this won't diminish any chances of experiencing a nightmare again as you sleep, it will allow you to receive answers, and will help put your mind at ease for the rest of the day.

Chapter 5

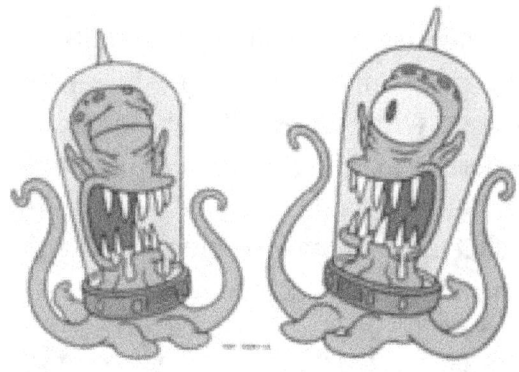

HOW TO TELL THE DIFFERENCE BETWEEN NIGHTMARES AND NIGHT TERRORS

While nightmares and night terrors, or parasomnias, have some features in common, they are different experiences. Nightmares have occurred when an individual awakens from a vivid dream with an intense feeling of fear and/or dread.

In contrast, night terrors are partial arousals from sleep during which an individual may shout, thrash their arms, kick, or scream. In addition, night terrors rarely occur in adults, while nightmares are experienced by people of all ages. Because nightmares and night terrors are two different types of sleep experiences, they should be differentiated and handled differently.

Learn the Traits Of A Nightmare

Nightmares are a type of undesirable sleep experience that can occur while you are falling asleep, sleeping, or waking up.

There are several characteristic features of experiencing a nightmare:

The storyline of the nightmare is often related to threats of your safety or survival. People experiencing nightmares will awake from their vivid dream with feelings of fear, stress, or anxiety. When the dreamers of nightmares wake up, they will often remember the dream, and be able to repeat the details. They will be able to think clearly upon awakening. Nightmares often keep the dreamer from falling back to sleep easily.

Expect Nightmares to Occur In People of All Ages

Nightmares are most common in children ages 3-6, with up to 50% of children experiencing nightmares during these ages. However, nightmares are often experienced by adults as well, especially if the individual is experiencing a particularly high amount of anxiety of stress.

Recognize When Nightmares Occur

Nightmares occur most often later in the sleep cycle during Rapid Eye Movement (REM) sleep. This is the period of time when dreaming is most prevalent, and it is when both good dreams and nightmares most commonly occur.

Consider Root Causes Of Nightmares

While nightmares can occur for no reason at all, seeing or hearing something that frightens or alarms a person can result in a nightmare. The sights or sounds that cause a nightmare can be things that have really happened, or things that are make-believe. Common causes of nightmares include illness, anxiety, the loss of a loved one, or a negative reaction to a medication, and Post-Traumatic Stress Disorder.

Prepare For The Aftermath Of Nightmares.

Nightmares usually leave the dreamer with intense feelings of fear, terror, and/or anxiety. It may be very difficult to return to sleep after a nightmare. Expect to console your child or love one after a nightmare. He or she may need to be calmed down and assured that there is nothing to be frightened of.

Adults, teens, or older children experiencing nightmares may benefit from speaking with a counselor who can help identify the source of stress, fear, or anxiety that is manifesting as nightmares.

Determine If A Person Is Likely To Experience Night Terrors.

While night terrors are relatively uncommon overall; they occur most often in children (experienced by up to 6.5% of children). Night terrors may be a consequence of the maturation of the central nervous system. By contrast, night terrors are rarely experienced by adults (only 2.2% of adults will experience night terrors). When adults experience night terrors, it is often due to underlying psychological factors such as trauma or stress.

Night terrors in children are usually not a cause for alarm. There is no evidence suggesting that a child who experiences night terrors has a psychological problem, or is upset about or disturbed by something. Children usually grow out of night terrors.

Night terrors do seem to have a genetic component. Children are more likely to experience night terrors if someone else in the family suffers from them as well.

Many adults who have night terrors also have another psychological condition, including bipolar disorder, depressive disorder, or an anxiety disorder.

Night terrors in adults can also be caused by post-traumatic stress disorder (PTSD), or by substance abuse (particularly alcohol abuse). It is crucial to consider potential underlying causes of night terrors in adults, and address these underlying causes if need be.

Indentify the Behaviors Associated With Night Terrors

There are certain behaviors that are often associated with night terrors. Common behaviors include:

Sitting up in bed

Screaming or shouting in fear

Kicking his or her feet

Thrashing his or her arms

Sweating, breathing heavily, or having a rapid pulse

Staring wide-eyed

Engaging in aggressive behavior (this is more common in adults that in children)

Recognize When Night Terrors Occur

Night terrors often occur during non-REM sleep, most commonly occurring during the short wave period of sleep. This means that they often will happen during the first few hours of sleep.

Don't Expect To Awaken a Person Having A Night Terror

People who are having a sleep terror episode will often be very hard to awaken. However, if they do awaken, they will often emerge from sleep in a confused state, and may be unsure why they appear to be sweaty, out of breath, or why their bed may be in disarray.

Expect the person to have no memory of the event. Occasionally people may recall vague information about the event, but there is no recollection of vivid detail. Even if you do manage to wake up the person, she/he will often be unaware of your presence, or be unable to recognize you.

Be Patient with the Person Experiencing the Night Terror

It is likely that he or she will have a difficult time communicating, even if she/he appears to be "awake" after the night terror occurs. This is because the night terror occurred during deep sleep.

Beware Of Dangerous Behaviors

A person having a night terror may pose a threat to him or herself, or to others without knowing it.

Watch out for sleepwalking. A person who is having a night terror can engage in sleepwalking, which can pose a serious threat.

Protect yourself from combative behavior. Abrupt physical movements (punching, kicking, and thrashing) often accompany sleep terrors and can cause injury to the person having a sleep terror, someone sleeping next to them, or someone attempting to control them.

How to Handle Night Terror

You should not attempt to wake up a person who is having a night terror unless she/he is in danger. Stay with the person having a night terror until she/he has calmed down.

Differentiating Between Nightmares and Night Terrors

1. Determine whether the person has woken up. A person who has a sleep terror episode will remain asleep, while someone who has a nightmare will wake up, and may remember vivid details about the dream.

2. See whether the person is easy to awaken. Someone who is having a nightmare can be easily awoken and brought out of the nightmare, but this is not the case with a night terror. In the case of the latter, the person will be extremely difficult to wake up, and may not actually emerge from their deep sleep.

3. Observe the state of the person after the episode. If the person who has experienced the episode appears confused, and is unaware of the presence of others in the room, s/he has likely experienced a night terror, and will often immediately return to sleep. On the other hand, if the person wakes up with feelings of fear or anxiety, and seeks out the comfort or company of another person (especially in the case of children) s/he has had a night mare. Remember that a person who has had a nightmare will often take longer to fall back to sleep.

4. Note when the episode occurs. If the episode occurs during the first few hours of sleep (most commonly

about 90 minutes after falling asleep), it most likely has occurred during the early short wave period of sleep. This indicates that the episode is probably a night terror. However, if the episode occurs later while in the sleep cycle, it most likely has occurred during REM sleep and is a nightmare.

Chapter 6

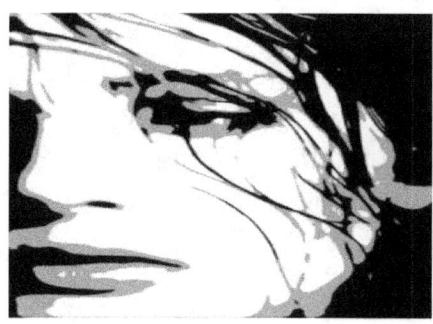

HOW TO STOP NIGHTMARES IN ADULTS

Nightmares run the range of strange to unsettling, to downright terrifying, often staying with us long after we have awaken. While it might be easy to write off a nightmare as something unimportant, nightmares (as well as dreams) are often windows into the subconscious mind. When nightmares become too much to handle, however, some proactive approaches are required to stop nightmares in adults. Occasional nightmares are a natural function of the brain, but if you feel like nightmares are taking over then these tips will help.

Nightmares cause physiological changes in the body that easily disturb a normal sleeping pattern. Many people wake up from nightmares in the middle of the night, and have difficulty going back to sleep. This is sometimes accompanied by an increased heart rate, sweating a feeling of anxiety, headache, and nausea. Overtime the imagery of nightmares begins slipping away as soon as someone wakes up, leading to sleepless nights trying to piece together what caused the reaction in the first place.

Nightmares often cause one to feel tired, groggy, irritable, and generally uncomfortable throughout the day. Waking up from a nightmare often causes mild confusion and disorientation that distracts from important tasks throughout the day. This is one of the primary reasons that it is important to stop nightmares in adults; something damaging occurring in sleep can affect work, family, and personal well-being in a long lasting way.

Nightmares are often caused by unresolved issues, so one of the first steps to stopping nightmares is to address those issues carefully. This include a wide range of behaviors such as addressing relationship issues, talking to someone else, creating lists of short and long term goals, seeing a therapist, and making general lifestyle changes. Some people find it helpful to keep a dream journal to identify patterns in nightmares.

For example, sometimes the content of nightmares is very clear; someone afraid of losing their home might have a nightmare about getting the foreclosure notice. In these cases it's easier to pinpoint the fear involved in the nightmare and strategically approach it. That person might not be able to suddenly produce money to secure their home, but they can plan, and take steps to feel more secure. More ambiguous nightmares may contain a wide range of images and sensations that are not specific or are difficult to remember. In these cases, seeing a therapist, or working, or reducing stress levels can help decrease the nightmares.

Reducing stress is one of the easiest ways for adults to stop nightmares. Meditation, yoga, exercise, massage, mindfulness techniques, and general time spent on self are all healthy ways to remove stress. When the body and mind are less stressed the chances of nightmares decrease. Changes in diet, or the usage of a sleeping supplement may also aid in getting rid of nightmares in adults. As always a comfortable bedroom area focused solely on sleep helps adults leave worries and issues behind, and focus on restful and satisfying sleep without nightmares.

How to Calm a Child Suffering From Night Terrors

The first key point is that night terrors are significantly different from nightmares. It is important to establish which your child is suffering from as the management, or treatment can be different depending on whether it is a nightmare or a night terror they are experiencing. Hug them if they will let you and talk soothingly without causing any further stress while they fall back asleep, is the most effective way to calm a child suffering from a sleep disorder.

Waking them up fully, screaming and panicking along with them are NOT the solution, and will only make things worse. Although it will seem like your child is awake, during a night terror children will appear confused, will be inconsolable and will likely not recognize you. This can be very distressing for the parent or other person witnessing the episode.

Nightmare or Night Terror

- o Night terrors occur during deep sleep in the first third of the night within a few hours of falling asleep, whereas nightmares more often occur in the morning.

- o Nightmares are more often remembered whereas night terror sufferers often have no recollection that anything happened at all (although some adults report seeing, spiders, tigers or shadowy figures).

- o Sufferers wake up from nightmares, but remain asleep throughout the night, and night terror sufferers are sleep even if they open their eyes! (Observers report sufferers sitting upright in bed, eyes wide open and screaming-scary stuff to watch).

- o Night terrors can cause the sufferer to experience an accelerated heart rate, sweating and confusion.

- o Night terror sufferers may sleep walk or thrash around so try to keep them safe.

Remember that you are not alone in having a child who suffers from a sleep disorder as there are estimates that as many as 15% of children suffer from them at some point, and many believe that this figure is under reported as many parents may dismiss the incidents as nightmares.

Occurrence is more common in boys than girls. Search the web for information, and you will find posts, blogs, and websites dedicated to sleep disorders and problems in children. Discussing issues is a proven way to reduce stress and discover coping mechanisms or solutions. Remember that terrors are most common in children aged between 2 and 6 years old, although they can occur at any age, and have been observed in kinds who are; overtired or ill, stressed, or fatigued; taking a new medication, sleeping in a new environment, or away from home.

So chances are that your child will grow out of these episodes, in fact they may only ever have one or they may suffer frequent attacks. There causes are unknown, but there are many theories ranging from eating a large meal before bedtime, psychic energy, developing brain, period of emotional conflict, tension or stress to certain medications. These are not what cause the terror; it simply allows your mind to be in a state in which a night terror is more likely to occur.

There is no known or proven treatment or cure (aside from some anecdotal evidence about EMF, and energy balancing products), but you can help prevent them:

1. Reduce your child's stress.

2. Establishing and sticking to a consistent bedtime routine that is simple and relaxing will help.

3. Make sure your child gets enough rest, let them nap during the day if necessary, or go to bed early if they are especially tired.

4. Prevent your child from becoming overtired by staying up too late.

5. A night terror, also known as a sleep terror or pavor nocturnes, is a parasomnia disorder characterized by extreme terror, and a temporary inability to regain full consciousness.

Understanding night terrors can reduce your worry-and help you get a good night's sleep yourself. But if night terrors continue for prolonged periods and happen repeatedly it would be wise to talk to your doctor about whether a referral to a sleep specialist is needed.

Chapter 7

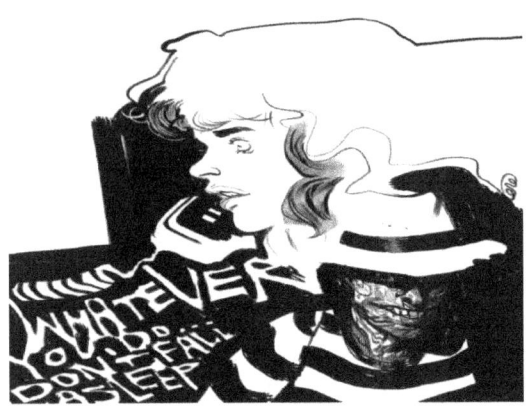

LEARN FROM YOUR NIGHTMARES
Face Your Nightmares

Nightmares show us what we are afraid of. What we are afraid of we are probably not dealing with. Just remembering a nightmare is the beginning of handling them. Your goal can be to handle your nightmares so that you can deal with them and what scares you in life.

How Nightmares Train You to Handle Your Fears

In life there are things that go wrong. We get sick. We get betrayed and deceived. We lose things. People die that are close to us. We love and lose. We can lose our job, our money, our friends, and our lives. Nightmares come to us, not just to warn us of a situation we may be creating, but to train us in dealing with the negative in life. If you can deal with the negative in dreams you can deal with the negatives in life.

A Nightmare Is Any Dream We Wake Up From In Fear

Why are we frightened in our dreams? Look at yourself in your nightmare and see how you are probably trying to hide or run from the dream situation, rather than facing it.

Example: this is a typical chase scene. Someone is chasing you in your dream, and you run thinking this figure chasing you will hurt you. However, as many dream work students have done, you can choose to turn around and face the chaser, and ask them what they want from you.

In life, face your adversaries the best you can, rather than run from them. Yet if the situation is overwhelming, sometimes the right choice is to flee.

A Nightmare Is Always Where the Image Of You In The Dream Feels Attacked Or Is Attacked

Just as in life, the "you in the dream" has unconscious attitudes. When in your next nightmare you feel afraid and overwhelmed, so much so you feel you have to wake yourself up, then after doing so, look at the attitude you had in the dream.

Attitudes DreamWorks: Is it something like, what I don't know will hurt me. Or, I am not strong enough to handle my life. Or, I will just make things worse if I confront this situation. There are many possible attitudes motivating our fears. Once you find the fear-attitudes that fit you, create the opposite attitude and use that attitude instead. For example, "I can deal with almost anything if I choose to". Next, rewrite your nightmare with the new attitude instead. Like, "I can deal with almost anything if I choose to".

Next, rewrite your nightmare with the new attitude and how you might act differently. This works very well also in training your children to handle their nightmares. Only you tell stories together, the original nightmare of your child, now turned into a positive "dealing with story".

Learn To Be More Heroic In Your Dreams, And You Will Be Heroic In Life In Dealing With Bad Things.

As in point 4, DreamWorks is doing something positive with your dream. With a series of nightmares you have you can rewrite each one in which you are acting more positively. Don't change the fear-inducing imagery, only your own attitude and behavior in the dream. If the dream imagery changes naturally, go with it.

Dream Example: a student had a repeat nightmare on several different nights in which this woman in the park near where she lived chased her. The faster she ran the faster the woman behind her ran. She shared this in dream group and was asked, why not stop in your dream and face the woman and ask what she wants? The next night she dreamed her chase dream again, but remembered to turn and asked the woman why she was chasing her. The chaser said she just wanted to catch up to her, and make friends with her!

The fundamental attitude here is to not assume a person or situation will do you harm. First accept the situation as it is and then find out its meaning and deal with it.

Find Out What You Are Afraid Of In Dreams

In your dream you may be afraid that things get out of control, and so your dream-creator creates a dream in which you are not able to control the situation. In dreams and life you may habitually resist others and situations not of your own choosing. This can show up in nightmares. Learn to accept things and not try to control them. Work with a person, or situation rather than try and dominate out of fear.

You may not be facing that your life behavior is dangerous, like driving too fast. Then you have a nightmare of crashing your car with enough intensity to scare you into facing the reality of how you do drive. When having a nightmare, find out what in the dream you are afraid of, and see if a similar situation is happening in you and your life.

Dream Example: Yes, this dream happens to people. A woman dreamed of driving her car going down a steep hill when she realized her brakes were not working. She woke herself up before she crashed. Yes, she had her car brakes checked, but she realized her attitude and behavior was that she was going too fast in her life. She had no brakes. She was not limiting herself and her compulsive behavior, and if she did not slow down, or take breaks, she would indeed crash, like sickness, car accident, losing a relationship, God knows what!

Use Your Dreams to Find Out What You Are Afraid Of In Life

Each nightmare represents a fear you have in life. If you are afraid you have cancer in life, or will get some terrible disease, then you may dream of that happening in a nightmare. Nightmares are also dreams that show us we lack the ability to control what happens to us. In life we are not heroes that can overcome any adversity. We don't have the power to control what happens to us. We do have some power to relate to the dark side of life through choice and available resources. Don't let fear paralyze you, or you will not deal with adversity as you can.

Dream-Life example: a teenage boy the author worked with in a treatment center dreamed he was swimming in the bay, and a giant hand reached up and pulled him under. After five years of residential treatment the boy did get better and go out on his own as a young adult. However, he wanted to go to Europe, and got into a cargo carrier box going to Europe. When they opened the box in Europe he was suffocated. This boy was still weak in his perception of reality, and could not protect himself in a real world. He dreamed his problem of going into dangerous places, in his mind or in outer life, and not pay attention to the real dangers of being overwhelmed. It took his life, just as surely as heavy drug addiction takes the lives of its users.

Fear Is Seeing What Could Happen That Is a Danger To You, But Not Actually Happening

Fear is perception of possible loss. The amazing thing is we all get afraid of things that could happen, but are not actually happening. Maybe a trauma happened to you in the past so you fear it happening again. The reality is more like good and bad things happen to us in life about equally. It's what we do with them that count. If we stay in fear, we try to run away, freeze up, or reject what might be life-enhancing because we are afraid it could go wrong. Our nightmares give us situations that may point this out to us. The solution is to deal with dangers realistically, and with all the strength we can summon to handle things. Teach your kids to do this also.

Know the difference between what is a real danger, and what is your projecting danger.

We Have No Time to Be Afraid

Think of situations in which you have been in danger. Did you just freeze up or did you do something? The reality point is that when in a dangerous situation don't project worse than it is, or you might freeze up. Accept what is happening, but relax, accept it as it is, and then you have more choice and power to do something, even if it is only to prevent worse from happening. Dreams can rehearse this kind of thing with us. Work on the scary dreams to get to a place where you rewrite, and relive them with you being as active as possible and not projecting worse into the situation as it actually happening.

Fear Is An Attitude And Not A Reality. We Have Nothing to Be Afraid Of In Life or In Our Dreams

Yes, we have nothing to be afraid of in life. We can be hurt, and probably will be. We can be killed by disease, accident, or criminality. But as long as we are alive and well, we are alive and well. Don't let attitudes that the worst will happen govern you living life now in each moment. Don't let negativistic attitudes control you in life. Dreams teach you this is you let them. Not only look at your nightmares or scary dreams. Look also at your positive dreams and learn from them. Now how did your dream have you solving that problem? Always look for something positive, even in the worst nightmare. Don't project it there. See it there. Change your attitude.

Dreams Mirror Life, Life Mirrors Our Dreams

We know that by now, don't we? When you remember a dream, ask yourself, how is that also happening in my life? It might not be the exact same content, but a similar content in which you react in a similar way. What's good at following our dreams when we remember them is that they teach us about ourselves. The first DreamWorks method is to look at how you are acting and not acting, and try to see why you act in the dream the way you do. Then ask yourself, how could I have acted more positively and effectively? Decide to do that next time in dreams or life in when such a situation comes up. As we change how we act in life for the better we will also be more effective in how we act in dreams. As in dreams, so in life!

To Fulfill yourself in Life Keep Extending the Circle of the Things You Are Not Afraid Of

We know this don't we? Those of us who are pretty much afraid all the time have a narrow limit of experiences. The more the variety of experiences we let ourselves have in life the more we learn how to cope with life and make the most of it. Thus when you are afraid to do something new, consider if maybe you can risk doing that new thing for the benefits you might gain. This doesn't mean you just unconsciously let go and jump off a cliff. Consider the risks, and consider doing what is an acceptable risk to you, and see what happens and see how it makes you a more effective person in dreams, in life, and in relationships. Remember, you are responsible for your own choices in life, and no one can make your choices for you. Having said this, then choose and deal with the consequences. Learn from life by living life.

Write Down Your Nightmares and Complete Them

A nightmare is an uncompleted dream that we wake up in fear from before the dream can complete itself.

Dream Example: Who knows, maybe when falling in a dream you should let yourself complete the fall and see what happens? So, when you wake up from a nightmare, write it down, and give it an ending that feels right for you and the dream. Make yourself stronger in the dream if necessary, and see what new dream imagery comes to you that resolves the dream situation. Then see how this completed dream is a lesson for you in how to better deal with life.

Use Allies in Your Dreams

Yes, some of us are able to be aware in some of our dreams to strengthen ourselves. If you can't do this it can be a nightmare itself, and then after waking up you can close your eyes and go back into the nightmare, but this time take a positive person, or power object with you to help you out. See what happens this time when you encounter the same nightmare situation.

Dream Example: A long-time student of her dreams had a positive figure show up in her depressing dreams. This figure gave her hope she was not alone. She learned in her depressing dreams to call on this helpful woman, dream figure to guide her through the darkness of her dreams. In life also, she successfully transformed into someone a lot more positive and able to deal with herself, her dreams, and the stresses of life.

Paint Your Nightmares, But Put A Golden Circle around That Figure You Are Afraid Of

Some people paint their dreams. You don't have to be an artist to do so. Just taking your child's crayons, or whatever, and putting marks on paper inspired by your dream can have emotional results for you. If you paint your fears, your darkness, your anger, evoked in you by a nightmare, or happening in your life, it releases your blocks. Colors often used for anger, or adversity, are black or red, or yellow. But if things feel really dark you can paint a healing symbol for you in your picture, or that of your child's. Or a golden circle. This helps balance the dark side coming out in your painting, and thus is more healing and balancing.

Look At Your Nightmares and Other Dreams for What Is Happening, or Not Happening in Your Intimate Relationships

For health's sake people in intimate relationships should be honest, expressive and very real. All involved should make it safe for each member of the relationship to express all the many sides of themselves. Thus, we have a lot of relating dreams, some of them nightmare or fear dreams. You can share some of your dreams in the relationship, but watch out because dreams are the most honest part of yourselves. They often reveal hidden thoughts and behavior concerning our relationships. Be committed to dealing fully and honestly with what is happening in relationship, even if first revealed in a dream.

Dream-Life Example: A woman dreamed her partner was having a relationship with another woman. That afternoon she asked her man if he was having an affair. He was honest and said yes. They chose to end their relationship. Thus, if you follow your dreams honestly, and share some of them in relationship it will make your relationship honest as well! It is more important that a relationship is fully real then it lasting a long time.

Your Fears Make You Stronger

An author was very afraid in some of his dreams and in life situations. He realized that fear means realness. He cannot fool himself. He cannot paint lovely pictures, and avoid the dangers in his life, or his inadequacies. So he turned his attitude around to face his fears, and thus build a better life.

How to Analyze Your Image in the Dream

DreamWorks Attitudes Technique: First, list what you are in the dream, and what your dream ego is doing in the dream or nightmare. Then try to think of an attitude motivating each of the actions you do in the dream. Then evaluate. Ask yourself; is my behavior and attitude appropriate to the dream situation, or off? If you are off, then you are incongruent. This means you are not in tune with what is happening.

Whether in a dream or life situation, such as in intimate relating, or at work, see if you are usually congruent with situations, in tune with them as they are, and cooperative in bringing out their value. When you find yourself in conflict, usually it is some attitude in you, such as, things should be fair, and that's blocking you from cooperative handling of the situation. Fairness is an attitude, not a truth. Things are often not fair in life, so deal with them as they are.

Find Out If You Live From Negative or Positive Motivation in Life

This is a great one! There are only two motivations for living life, positive or negative, or some combination of both.

Life Value: Either I live from fear, needing to be secure, needing to control people and things, or I live from the creative, the opposite and fear. A creative person accepts most of a situation and chooses to develop the values possible therein. They accept, and then see what is positive that can come out of the situation, and they emphasize that, while still dealing with the negatives, but not exaggerating them. Look for these two motivational attitudes in your dreams and in your behavior.

Choose To Be Positive and Accepting In Dreams and Life and See How Things Go Better For You

Finally, when you have insights about yourself, others, and life they mean little if you don't act upon them. If you are caught in a negative motivation; try to start to do things from positive motivation. See what happens for you. Also, try to limit your negative attitudes, at least pause, and see if you can choose to be positive in the situation. Look in your dreams for positive things you do, and see how you can do these things also in life.

Transform yourself and your nightmares at the same time.

Conclusion

Thank you again for choosing this book!

These are methods to confronting and putting an end to a nightmare and night terror. In addition, it is known that escaping from a nightmare is how many people initially start learning how to lucid dream. Escaping from the nightmares can trigger lucidity, potentially allowing you to naturally lucid dream, freely keeping a regular wake-sleep schedule are important. So is engaging in regular exercise, which will help alleviate nightmare-causing anxiety and stress. You may find that yoga and meditation are also helpful.

Remember to practice good sleep hygiene, which will help prevent the sleep deprivation that can bring on nightmares in adults. Make your bedroom a relaxing, tranquil place that is reserved for sleep, so you don't associate it with stressful activities.

Also, be cautious about the use of alcohol, caffeine, and nicotine, which can remain in your system for more than 12 hours, and often disrupt sleep patterns.

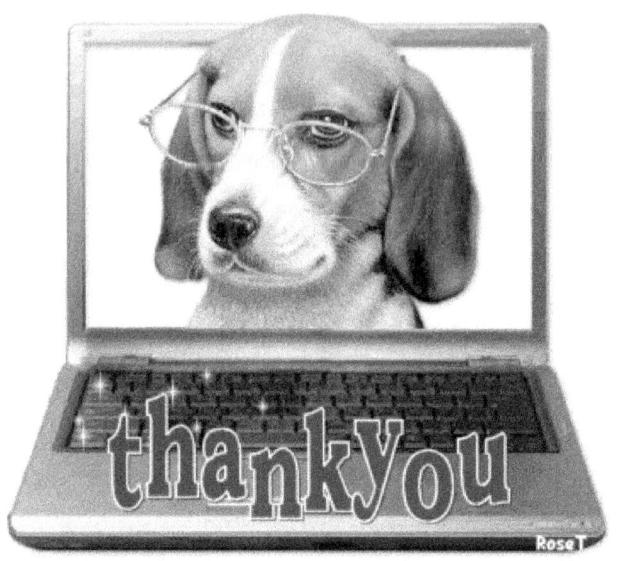

Finally, if you enjoyed this book, would you be kind enough to leave a review for this book on Amazon? It'd be greatly appreciated!

Thank you and good luck!

Preview Of 'NIGHT TERRORS IN CHILDREN: LEARN HOW TO BATTLE NIGHT TERRORS IN CHILDREN'

Chapter 1

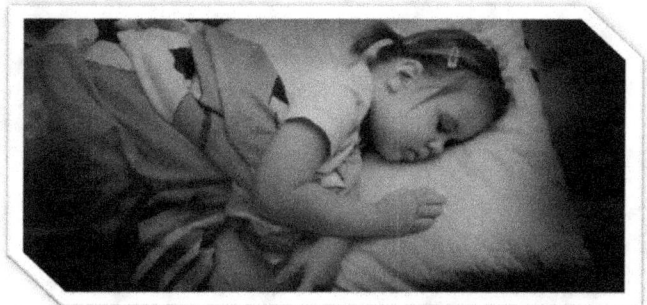

WHAT ARE NIGHT TERRORS

Night terrors are sleep disturbances in which a child may suddenly bolt upright in bed, cry, scream, and moan, mumble, and thrash about with his or her eyes wide open, but without being truly awake. Because they are caught in a sort of a twilight zone between being asleep and being awake, they're unaware of your presence and isn't likely to respond to anything you say or do.

In fact, researchers think of night terrors as mysterious glitches in the usually smooth transitions we make each night between sleep stages. As many as 6 percent of children have night terrors at some point, typically beginning in the toddler and preschool, years and continuing up to age 7 or even adolescence.

An episode can last anywhere from five to 45 minutes, and when it's over your child falls back to sleep abruptly with no memory of the incident.

How are night terrors different from nightmares?

Unlike a night terror, a nightmare leaves your child truly awake – he or she can remember their dream and sometimes talk about it, and they seek out and feel comforted by your presence.

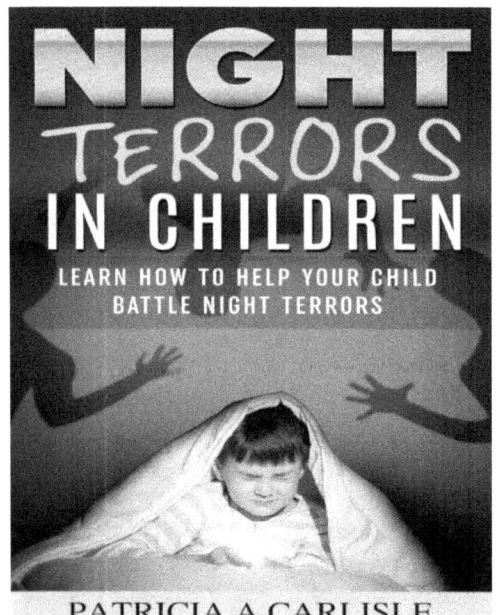

To check out the rest of (NIGHT TERRORS IN CHILDREN: LEARN HOW TO HELP YOUR CHILD BATTLE NIGHT TERRORS) go to Amazon.com

Check Out My Other Books

Below you'll find some of my other popular books that are popular on Amazon and Kindle as well. Alternatively, you can visit my author page on Amazon to see other work done by me.

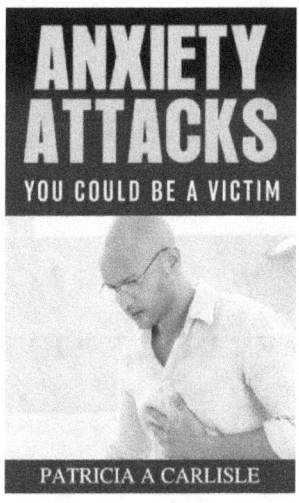

ANXIETY ATTACKS: YOU COULD BE A VICTIM.

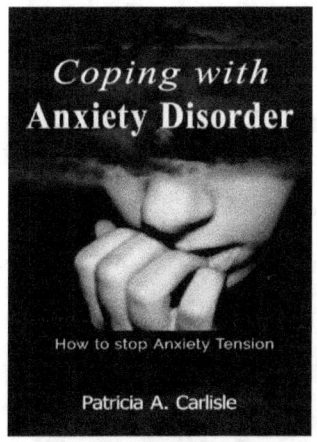

COPING WITH ANXIETY DISORDER: HOW TO STOP ANXIETY TENSION.

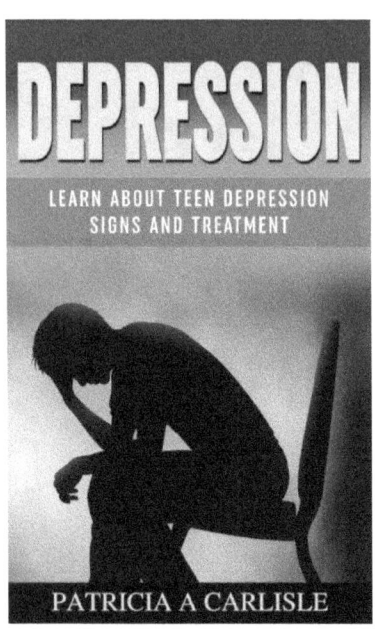

DEPRESSION: LEARN ABAOUT TEEN DEPRESSION SIGNS AND TREATMENT.

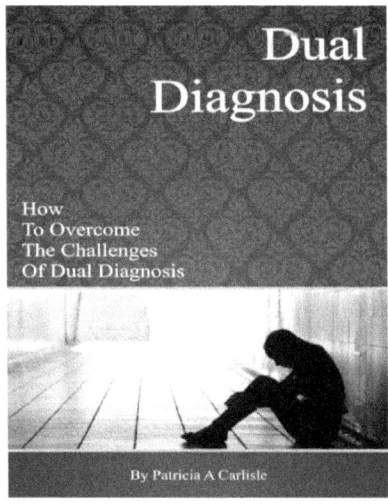

DUAL DIAGNOSIS: HOW TO OVERCOME THE CHALLENGES OF DUAL DIAGNOSIS.

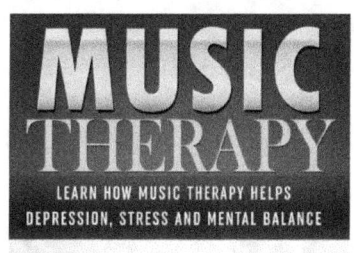

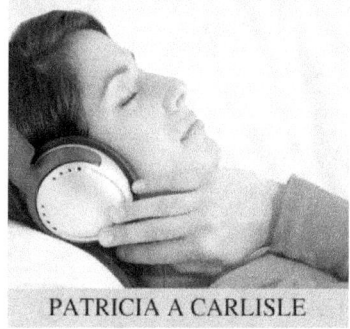

MUSIC THERAPY: LEARN HOW MUSIC THERAPY HELPS DEPRESSION, STRESS AND MENTAL BALANCE.

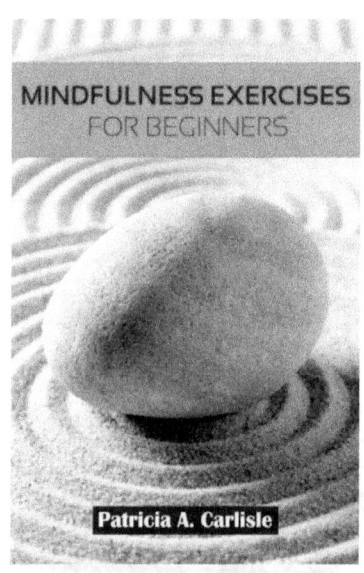

MINDFULNESS EXERCISES FOR BEGINNERS.

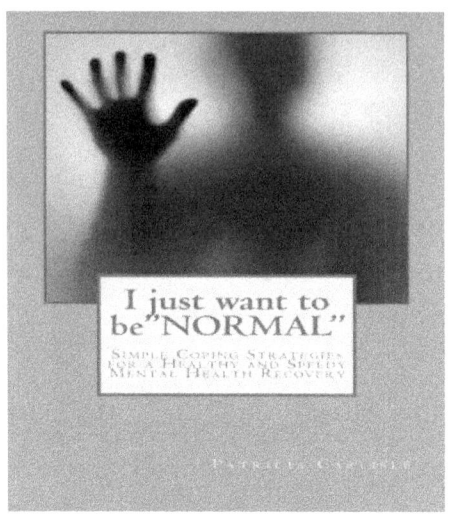

I just want to be "NORMAL" Simple Coping Strategies for a Healthy and Speedy Mental Health Recovery.

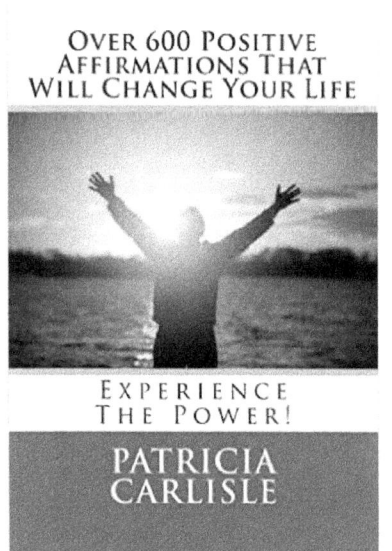

OVER 600 POSITIVE AFFIRMATIONS THAT WILL CHANGE YOUR LIFE. EXPERIENCE THE POWER!

BONUS: SUBSCRIBE TO THE FREE BOOK

Beginners Guide to Yoga & Meditation

"Stressed out? Do You Feel Like The World Is Crashing Down Around You? Want To Take A Vacation That Will Relax Your Mind, Body And Spirit? Well this Easy To Read Step By Step

E-Book Makes It All Possible!"

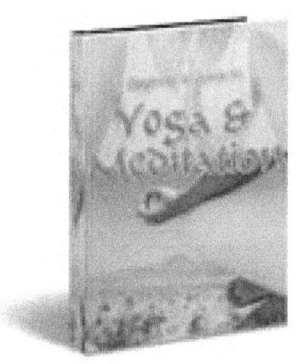

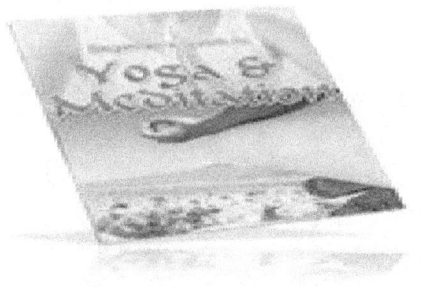

Instructions on how to join our mailing list, and receive a free copy of "Yoga and Meditation" can be found in any of my Kindle eBooks.

NOTES

NOTES

NOTES

NOTES

NOTES

www.ingramcontent.com/pod-product-compliance
Lightning Source LLC
Chambersburg PA
CBHW071245280526
45788CB00004B/1589